A Whole New You:
How I Got Back My Desired Body In 41 Days.

Lewis Green

Table of Contents

Introduction

All across the world, people are struggling with stubborn body fats.
Just like me. You don't have to be one of them anymore!

In my book, I will share my personal experience, step by step, on how I got back get back my 48 kg body from 80 kg.

By following my easy steps, you will get back a body you're proud to show off on the beach in 41 days!

Furthermore, as a bonus, I will also teach you:

The basics on how to prepare meals that you and your family will surely love without having to gaining a single pound.

My own simple juicing recipes that not only help you lose weight but also a body detoxing aid.

And many more...on my journey in getting back my slim and attractive body.

My Story

My story starts off like many others. I once thought of myself as overweight and unattractive because I had too much fat on my body. I never wanted to show my skin in public, and I definitely never saw myself going to the beach again. I knew that if I ever wanted to look good in a bathing suit, I was going to have to do something about my weight. Unfortunately, every diet plan I ever tried failed, and I had no idea how to work out the right way or what I should be eating to make a difference in my appearance.

It did not help that I had two children, and I never was completely able to lose the weight I had gained while pregnant. Unfortunately, as time went on, I found it harder and harder to find a chance to prepare healthy meals or get to the gym. Now that I had a growing family, I knew I was never going to be able to make the kinds of changes in my life that I needed to do in order to lose weight fast.

Finally, I realized that it might be easier than I thought to drop back down to the size I was before I ever had children. Why would I need to spend time every day for the rest of my life trying to fit in a complicated diet plan or lengthy workout routine if I could just make a few changes and lose weight fast? I set out to create the perfect diet and exercise plan to get myself in shape and help drop the weight fast. Now, I am here to share this plan with you.

If you follow my diet and workout tips, you will be able to lose weight in less than six weeks. Stick to the plan for 41 days and you will soon find yourself shedding your weight and feeling better than ever. It takes a little bit of willpower and just a small amount of extra time every day, but if you follow my tips, you will have no trouble making the kinds of changes you need in your life and losing weight fast.

The best part of my diet plan is that you do not have to be a world-class chef to prepare the simple, healthy recipes outlined here. When you cook these delicious meals, your whole family will want to join you in your diet plan, and you will not have to waste a ton of time in the kitchen every day either. Pair these tasty dishes and excellent juice recipes with a simple workout program and you will shed weight quickly and keep it off easily. Read on to find out more about the diet and exercise plan that changed my life!

What Makes Food Healthy?

There are many different types of food groups that you should eat when you are looking to supplement your diet with the best possible nutrients. On the other hand, there are several groups of food that you should avoid if you hope to lose weight and keep it off. Read up on the following tips to discover which foods are best and which ones you should stay away from while on your 41-day diet challenge.

Foods to Eat

Fill up on these healthy foods in order to provide the most benefit to your body on a daily basis.

Fruits and Vegetables. Fruits and veggies include plenty of vitamins and nutrients, and many also contain fiber, potassium, calcium, and a wide variety of other important factors for your health. Different colored fruits and vegetables contain different vitamins, so try to consume a wide variety of colors every day.

Omega3 Fatty Acids. Omega3 fatty acids are a type of unsaturated fat that can help reduce your risk of heart disease and improve your joint function. Be sure to eat plenty of fish and other seafood in order to get as many of these important nutrients as possible. Omega3 fatty acids are also said to be good at helping improve mood and emotional disorders such as depression.

Monounsaturated Fats. This type of fat can help lower your cholesterol and even help you control your blood sugar to a certain extent. You can find monounsaturated fats in olives and olive oil, avocados, nuts, and nut butter. Be sure to cook your meats in olive oil whenever possible in order to get a healthy amount of monounsaturated fats in your daily diet.

Whole Grains. If you are trying to avoid gluten, you do not have to consume whole grains, and should instead opt for flour and other traditionally grain-based foods that are made from nuts and seeds instead. If you are not avoiding gluten, however, be sure to cut bleached foods out of your diet, and stick to whole grains. White rice, white bread, and bleached pastas are difficult to digest and may cause stomach upset, where whole grains contain healthy nutrients.

Foods to Avoid

Trans Fats. Stay away from trans fats, which have been hydrogenated and which are known to raise bad cholesterol levels while simultaneously lowering good cholesterol levels. Trans fats have been linked to heart disease, diabetes, stroke, and even in some cases to cancer. Avoid them at all costs. Trans fats are found in packaged products, pre-made mixes, and solid fat sources like sticks of butter or margarine. Not all packaged products contain trans fats, so be sure to read your labels.

Corn Syrup. Although a small amount of natural sugar is fine in your food, and in fact your body does need a little bit of sugar every day, it is important to cut back significantly on your sugar intake in order to lose weight. Be sure to get your sugar from a healthy source, such as raw organic honey, rather than from processed corn syrup.

Vegetable Oil. Unfortunately, vegetable oil is a frequent cause of digestive upset in many dieters who do not know better than to keep eating this food. Remove it from your diet and replace it with much healthier olive or coconut oil instead. Vegetable oil can cause inflammation in your joins and even lead to heart disease when consumed too frequently.

How to Stock a Healthy Kitchen

Keep a healthy kitchen stocked at all times to make your food preparation that much easier! You should have no trouble whipping up a quick, easy, and very healthy meal or snack when you make sure to have all the necessary basics on hand every time you step into your kitchen. Remember that healthy eating starts at home, and that it is always better to prepare your meals yourself rather than going out to eat. If you find yourself lacking in some of the important items listed below, be sure to stock up before you get started on your 41-day diet challenge!

Utensils and Cookware

Keep the following utensils and cookware on hand at all times to make food preparation a breeze.

Pots. Pots and sauce pans are a must have for any kitchen. You can cook a lot of healthy dishes in a pot, including tasty soups and healthy chilies that are perfect for cold nights when you want to curl up with some comfort food.

Skillets. Use a skillet to fry up healthy alternatives to many of your favorite foods. Just about anything can be prepared in a skillet, which makes this a versatile member of your kitchen team. It is a good idea to have at least two skillets of different sizes available, for those times when you need to prepare your main course and your side dish alongside each other on the stove top.

Cast iron skillet. It is always a good idea to have at least one large cast iron skillet around, particularly for those times when you need to prepare something partially on the stove and partially in the oven. Cast iron skillets can safely transfer between the two, and they can provide a lot of flavor when cooking meats and vegetables.

Casserole dish. Grab a casserole dish or a glass baking pan for those times when you want to make healthy lasagnas and other low-calorie baked foods. Add a loaf pan if you hope to make delicious healthy breads and sweet treats.

Healthy Ingredients

Stock up on these healthy ingredients to reach for the next time you are cooking something in your healthy kitchen.

Spices. Keep plenty of spices on hand to season your food and make it delicious. Dill, tarragon, cumin, black pepper, herbs de Provence, and cinnamon are all excellent choices. Be sure to use plenty of ginger in your cooking to aid in digestive health.

Nonfat milk or soy milk. When baking, you will need to have healthy milk alternatives available. Keep either nonfat dairy milk or soy milk on hand to make cooking even easier. You can also try almond milk if you have an allergy to soy or otherwise prefer to avoid it.

Olive oil. Olive oil is one of the healthiest alternatives when it comes to cooking food in a fat source. Use it in place of vegetable oil, or choose coconut oil for the healthiest option around. Olive oil keeps for a long time, which makes it a great choice for stocking up on early.

Raw organic honey or agave nectar. Keep these sugar sources on hand to substitute for real sugar or artificial sweeteners in your coffee, tea, and baking. Remember to calculate appropriately when you plan to use honey instead of sugar in baking recipes. With the right changes, you can have a delicious dessert that is much better for your body than it would be with processed sugar included.

How Juicing Helps

Juicing is an excellent way to supplement your diet with healthy drinks that can fill you up and give you tons of energy without adding a lot of calories to your daily intake. Best of all, if you purchase a juicer, you can easily process your ingredients and prepare fresh juices in almost no time right in your own kitchen.

Try out juicing as a part of your diet plan today, and consider adding a juicing detox to the beginning or end of your 41-day diet challenge. I planned a juicing detox at the end of my challenge, and it made a world of difference in helping me stay fit and stick to my diet in the future!

What Makes Juicing So Healthy?

Fruits and vegetables are packed with important vitamins and nutrients. When you process them through a juicer or blend them in a blender, you are exposing all of the inner portions of fruits and vegetables, which makes them much healthier and easier to eat. If you do not add any extra ingredients to your juices, you can enjoy only the good parts of your vegetables and fruits, with no unnecessary sugars, fats or other problem foods. Most juice recipes are meant to be prepared without sugars, but if you like, you can always add a little bit of organic raw honey or agave nectar to sweeten your juices in a healthy way.

Juicing as a Dietary Supplement

One of the biggest reasons why juicing works so well as a dietary supplement is that it helps you reach your daily fruit and vegetable goals easily, without having to find a way to prepare several servings of these important food groups. You can select fruits and vegetables of many different colors in order to provide your body with tons of much-needed vitamins, all through the power of healthy juicing!

Although juicing is an excellent way to get plenty of nutrients on a daily basis, remember that it is still important to eat your fruits and vegetables now and then as well. When you process juices in your juicer, they do lose some of their beneficial qualities. They lose their pulp, which is where all of the fiber in these healthy treats is located. If you are looking to add more fiber to your diet, juicing may not be right for you. However, if you can get your fiber from other sources or be sure to eat vegetables along with your dinners, juicing is a great way to load up on healthy foods on the go.

Juicing Detox How-To

It is very important to follow a juicing detox plan that is designed to keep your body healthy and full of the nutrients it needs to function properly throughout the detox. Follow these steps to safely perform a juicing detox either before or after your diet. Again, I recommend doing this at the end of your 41 days!

Before: Three Days

Stick to your standard diet for three days, but be sure to drink at least 8 glasses of water every day. Cut back significantly on fats and sugars if you have not done this already. Do not consume coffee, soda, or alcohol. Drink only water, and occasionally caffeine-free herbal tea with nothing added to it.

Detox

You can plan your juicing detox for as long or as short a time as you feel is necessary. Most first-timers detox for three days, but five or seven day cleanses are appropriate as well. During your detox, drink a glass of water with lemon every morning, and then consume six different types of juice throughout the day. Drink one juice every two hours between the time you wake up and when you go to bed.

After: Three Days

After you have finished your detox, you will need to slowly work you way back up to eating solid foods again. Do not overload your system with food right away, as this can make you very sick. On the first day, eat fruits and vegetables along with eight glasses of water. On the second day, add nuts and any grains that do not contain gluten. On the final day, add meat and remaining grains. Your detox is now complete!

Weight Loss Workouts

Working out can make a huge difference in your diet plan. It is important to follow a simple workout schedule in order to make this 41-day challenge as successful as possible.

Best Weight Loss Workouts

There are two different types of workouts that you need to consider when trying to lose weight: cardio and strength training. Most of the time, cardio provides the best chance to burn calories quickly and lose weight fast. However, strength training has its merits, and if you work up to combining both in your weekly workout, you have the best possible chance of losing weight fast. Try these routines to see what worked best for me during my 41-day weight loss challenge.

Cardio: Running

One of the easiest ways to get your cardio exercise in is to just run for it! Running is simple and only requires a comfortable pair of shoes and a little bit of time. If you have a safe place to run in your neighborhood, you can easily make a ten-minute run a part of your routine after dinner every evening, or in the mornings before you go to work.

Cardio: Elliptical

If you have access to a gym or your own home elliptical machine, this can be an added bonus when it comes to cardio workouts. Use an elliptical slowly at first, and build up your resistance and your speed over time. It is important not to push yourself too hard at first when you are using one of these machines. If you do not have access to an elliptical, you can replace this part of the workout routine with uphill running or jogging up and down stairs.

Strength: Push-ups

If you are new to strength training, push-ups are a great place to start. Hold yourself up with your toes and wrists, and bend your elbows outward as you lower your body as far as possible before picking yourself up again. Repeat this process as many times as you can, but do not be discouraged if you can only do a few push-ups at first! You will work your way up to more in no time.

Strength: Crunches

Crunches are one of the simplest types of strength training, but they are an excellent way to shed weight quickly. Lie down on your back with your knees up and your arms crossed over your chest. Pick up your upper body as if you were doing a sit-up. If you find that you have trouble not lifting your feet off of the ground, ask someone to hold your feet for you, or hook them under a heavy chair or sofa to keep yourself from moving.

Weekly Routine

As a beginner to working out, you should follow this simple weekly routine to help lose weight fast. Make it a part of your 41-day challenge and be sure to stick to the schedule in order to get the most out of your exercise plan. You will only need a little bit of time out of your week to make this routine work, and you do not have to leave home to do any of it!

Day One: Cardio
Stretch first, then jog for 10 minutes.
Increase your speed and run for 5 minutes.
Decrease your speed and jog for 5 minutes more.
Stretch again to cool down.

Day Two: Rest

Day Three: Strength
Stretch first, then do 10 push-ups.
Do 10 crunches.
If you have enough endurance, repeat the process. Work up to repeating the process three times total.
Stretch again to cool down.

Day Four: Rest

Day Five: Cardio + Strength
Stretch first, then do 10 push-ups.
Jog for 10 minutes.
Increase speed, then run for 5 minutes.
Decrease speed, then jog for 5 minutes more.
Do 10 crunches.
Stretch again to cool down.

Day Six: Rest

Day Seven: Rest

Tips for Working Out

- Always stretch before and after you work out. This can reduce the risk of workout related injuries.

- Do not force yourself to do more than your body can handle during one workout. However, if you feel like you can go further than you used to, this means it is time to add more to your routine.

- You do not need complicated equipment or a lot of time to work out every day of the week. Set aside 20 to 30 minutes for three days per week to work out, and you will find great results in no time.

- In order to perform cardio and strength exercises at home, you only need a comfortable pair of running shoes and some clothes that are easy to move in.

- Listen to music while working out to make the time pass quickly!

Healthy Recipes

Try out these delicious healthy recipes to make your whole family happy! You will forget you are on a diet at all when you chow down on these delicious meals, snacks, and more.

Breakfast

Try these breakfast recipes for the perfect morning meal!

Avocado Muffin Sandwich

2 whole wheat English muffins, toasted

1 sliced avocado

2 tsp whole grain mustard

2 boiled eggs

Pinch of fresh dill

Cut boiled eggs into slices along with avocado.

Spread mustard onto each half of English muffin.

Top with sliced eggs, sliced avocado, and fresh dill.

Serves 2.

Scrambler

3 tsp olive oil

4 eggs

½ cup canned white beans with no sodium added

½ cup halved grape tomatoes

4 slices toasted bread

¼ cup jarred pesto

Salt and pepper to taste

Rinse canned beans thoroughly.

In a large bowl, beat eggs together with salt, pepper, and 1 tbsp water.

In a large skillet, heat 2 tsp oil over medium-high, then add beans and tomatoes. Cook for 2 minutes.

Remove from skillet, then heat remaining oil. Add eggs and cook for 2 minutes, stirring.

Serve scrambled eggs topped with beans. Finish with a spoonful of pesto and a side of toast.

Serves 2.

Banana Bread

¼ cup organic honey

6 tbsp applesauce, no sugar added

2 eggs

2 tbsp dark brown sugar

¼ cup unsweetened almond milk

3 large bananas

1 tsp vanilla extract

1 tsp baking soda

1-1/2 cups wheat flour

½ tsp cinnamon

Mash bananas to form around 1-1/2 cups of mashed banana.

Grease a loaf pan or spray with nonstick cooking spray.

Preheat oven to 325 degrees F.

Stir together applesauce with honey and brown sugar in a large mixing bowl.

Beat eggs into mixture well.

Add almond milk and mashed bananas, then stir to combine.

Add vanilla, baking soda, and cinnamon. Stir to blend until smooth.

Fold flour into banana mixture, but do not over-mix.

Pour batter into loaf pan. Bake for 1 hour, then cool for 10 minutes.

Slice and serve.

Poached Eggs

1 tbsp olive oil

2 tsp white vinegar

Dash black pepper

Dash salt

2 sliced tomatoes

8 eggs

1 tbsp thyme

1 oz shaved Parmesan cheese

4 slices bread, toasted

1 pound mushrooms, washed and sliced

2 tbsp chopped chives

In a large skillet with deep sides, bring 3 inches of water to a simmer with vinegar.

In a separate skillet over medium-high heat, cook tomatoes for 2 minutes per side, and season with salt and pepper.

Remove tomatoes to a plate. In the same skillet over medium-high heat, add mushrooms, salt, pepper, and thyme. Cook for 7 minutes, tossing.

While mushrooms cook, crack four eggs and gently slide into simmering vinegar water.

Cook eggs for 3 minutes, then remove with slotted spoon. Repeat for the other eggs.

Serve bread topped with tomatoes, eggs, mushrooms, cheese, and chives.

Serves 4.

Yogurt Parfait

2 tbsp organic almond butter

1 tbsp organic honey

¾ cup plain Greek yogurt, nonfat

3 strawberries

¼ cup grapes

2 tbsp chopped almonds

Slice grapes into halves; quarter strawberries.

In a small bowl, whisk yogurt together with almond butter and honey.

Serve in a glass, layering yogurt, grapes, strawberries, and almonds, and then repeat the layering once more.

Serves 1.

Lunch

Make your lunch much more exciting and healthy too with these simple meals.

Curry Chicken Salad

1 cup chopped pre-cooked bagged chicken breast strips

¼ cup nonfat mayonnaise

2 tsp water

1 tsp yellow curry powder

Dash salt

1/3 cup diced celery

1 cup chopped apple

3 tbsp golden raisins

In a large bowl, combine mayonnaise with water and curry until blended and smooth.

Toss with remaining ingredients until everything is coated in curry sauce mixture.

Cover and chill for at least 2 hours before serving.

Spelt Bean Salad

2-1/2 cup water

1-1/4 cup uncooked rinsed and drained spelt

½ cup parsley

½ cup mint

½ cup minced red onion

2 tbsp olive oil

3 tbsp lemon juice

Salt and pepper to taste

15 oz canned drained and rinsed navy beans

14oz canned drained and chopped artichoke hearts

In a medium pot over medium-low heat, bring spelt and water to a boil.

Cover and turn heat to low; simmer for 30 minutes, then stir.

In a large bowl, combine cooked spelt with remaining ingredients.

Cover and chill at least 2 hours in the refrigerator.

Serve.

BLT

1 tbsp minced onion

2 tbsp light mayonnaise

½ tsp minced sage

2 tsp Dijon

2 oz sliced pancetta

4 sliced tomatoes

8 slices toasted sourdough

1 cup arugula, washed and torn

In a large bowl, combine onions with mayonnaise, mustard, and sage. Stir until mixed thoroughly.

Preheat oven to 400 degrees F.

In a single layer on a cookie sheet, bake pancetta for 8 minutes, then drain.

Spread bread with mayonnaise mixture and top with 2 slices pancetta, 2 slices tomato, and arugula.

Serves 4.

Pasta Salad

2 cups shredded pre-cooked bagged chicken breast strips

½ pound uncooked penne pasta

½ cup sharp cheddar cheese, shredded

1 cup frozen corn

½ cup diced red pepper

½ cup diced green onion

½ cup diced tomato

2 tbsp lime juice

¼ cup orange juice

1 tbsp olive oil

1 tbsp chopped chili in adobo

Pinch salt

Cook pasta according to the directions on the package.

Drain pasta, then place in a large bowl with chicken, corn, cheese, pepper, onions, and tomato. Toss to combine flavors well.

In a small bowl, whisk together orange juice with oil, chilies, salt, and lime juice.

Pour mixture over pasta, then toss to combine all flavors well.

Cover and chill in the refrigerator for at least 2 hours.

Serve.

Avocado Soup

2 large chopped avocados

2 cups fat free low-sodium chicken broth

1 cup navy beans, rinsed and drained from can

1 cup water

1-1/2 tbsp lemon juice

½ cup nonfat plain yogurt

Salt and pepper to taste

Tabasco sauce to taste

1 seeded and chopped jalapeno pepper

1oz crumbled queso fresco

In a blender, combine all ingredients except cheese.

Puree on high until smooth and combined.

Scrape sides of blender, and place avocado mixture into four separate bowls.

Top with cheese and serve cold, or heat in microwave if you prefer your soup warm.

Serves 4.

Dinner

Dinner does not have to be difficult when you try these tasty creations!

Barbecue Chicken Potato

½ cup nonfat sour cream

4 baking potatoes

1-1/3 cup shredded pre-packaged barbecue chicken

2 chopped green onions

2oz nonfat shredded cheddar cheese

Wash potatoes and pierce all over skin with a fork.

Bake potatoes in oven at 400 degrees F for 1 hour. If you are short on time, microwave potatoes for 10 minutes on high, turning halfway through.

Combine sour cream with chopped green onions.

Microwave chicken on high for 2 minutes or until hot.

Serve potatoes sliced and topped with chicken, sour cream, and cheese.

Serves 4.

Cumin Chicken

4 boneless skinless chicken breasts

Dash salt

¾ tsp ground cumin

¾ cup shredded Mexican cheese, low-fat

10oz canned diced tomatoes and green chilies

2 tbsp cilantro, fresh

Preheat the broiler on your oven.

In a large cast iron skillet over medium-high heat, cook chicken for 6 minutes per side until done. Season with salt and cumin.

Remove cooked chicken from pan and add ¼ tsp cumin and canned, undrained tomatoes to skillet.

Add chicken again, and spoon mixture over all.

Sprinkle with cheese and broil for 2 minutes.

Serve topped with cilantro.

Serves 4.

Easy Chili

2 tsp chili powder

Sliced green onions to taste

Nonfat sour cream to taste

1 pound ground lean beef

14oz canned beef broth, no sodium added

14oz canned chili-seasoned tomato sauce

14oz frozen black bean and corn blend

In a large cast iron skillet or Dutch oven, combine chili powder and beef.

Cook and stir for 6 minutes over medium-high heat until beef is crumbled.

Drain and place beef mixture back into pan.

Add frozen corn mixture, tomato sauce, and broth, and bring to a boil.

Cover and turn heat to low. Simmer for 10 minutes, then uncover and simmer for 5 minutes more.

Serve topped with onions and sour cream.

Tropical Ham Quesadillas

4 multigrain tortillas

½ cup jarred mango chutney

½ cup crumbled queso fresco

8oz shaved deli ham with low sodium

3 tbsp chopped green onions

Preheat a grill to medium-high, or use a grill pan on your stovetop.

On each tortilla, spread 2 tbsp chutney and top with cheese, ham, and onions.

Fold in half and place onto grill rack.

Grill for 3 minutes per side.

Cut into wedges and serve.

Serves 4.

Stuffed Chile Poblanos

16oz canned refried beans, low sodium

½ cup jarred picante sauce

8oz microwavable rice pouch

4oz shredded nonfat Mexican cheese

4 chile poblano peppers

Cilantro to taste

Halve chile poblano peppers and remove seeds and membranes.

Place halves with the cut sides up on a microwave-safe plate, then cover with wax paper.

Microwave on high for 3 minutes.

Meanwhile, in a large bowl stir together picante sauce, beans, and rice.

When chilies have microwaved, fill with bean mixture.

Cover with wax paper and microwave on high for 2 minutes.

Sprinkle with cheese, then microwave on high for 2 minutes more.

Serve topped with cilantro.

Serves 4.

Wine Glazed Scallops

1 tbsp olive oil

1-1/2 tsp chopped tarragon

½ cup dry white wine

1 tbsp butter

Dash salt

Dash black pepper

1-1/2 pounds large fresh sea scallops

Dry scallops with a paper towel.

In a large skillet over medium-high heat, add oil and warm.

Cook scallops in oil for 3 minutes per side, then remove to a platter.

In the same skillet, add salt, tarragon, and wine, then scrape the bottom of the pan to remove any flavorful pieces that have cooked on.

Boil mixture for 1 minute, then remove from the heat.

Add butter and stir until melted.

Serve scallops topped with glaze and sprinkled with pepper.

Serves 4.

Grilled Chops

½ tsp black pepper

¼ tsp salt

¼ tsp ground allspice

¾ tsp cinnamon

¼ tsp ground cumin

1/8 tsp red pepper flakes

8 trimmed lamb chops

Prepare grill to medium-high heat. Alternately, use a grill pan on your stove, or turn your broiler to high.

Combine all spices in a small bowl, then rub chops evenly with spice mixture.

Grill for 5 minutes per side on grill or in grill pan. If broiling, broil for 5 to 7 minutes per side or until done.

Serve.

Serves 4.

Snacks

Snack on some of these simple and light bites to make your diet go smoothly.

Homemade Hummus

¼ cup lemon juice

5 tbsp water

3 tbsp olive oil

¼ cup tahini

Dash salt

1 crushed clove of garlic

2 (15oz) canned rinsed and drained chick peas

½ tsp paprika

1 tbsp toasted pine nuts

Fresh chopped parsley to taste

In a large food processor or blender, combine water, lemon juice, olive oil, tahini, salt, olive oil, garlic, and chick peas.

Puree on high until smooth.

Serve in a bowl topped with parsley, paprika, and parsley along with pita chips and vegetable spears.

Quick Guacamole

1 tbsp lime juice

1-1/2 tbsp chopped red onion

Pinch salt

1 clove garlic

1 peeled avocado with pit removed

½ small jalapeno pepper with stem removed

1 tbsp fresh cilantro leaves

In a blender or food processor, combine red onion, salt, lime juice, clove, and jalapeno pepper.

Pulse until chopped, then add avocado.

Blend on high until smooth.

Serve with cilantro sprinkled on top.

Caramel Cookie Bites

1 cup and 2 tbsp packed brown sugar

½ cup and 2 tbsp softened unsalted butter

2 tbsp milk

1 egg

1-1/2 cups gluten free flour

¾ tsp vanilla extract

Pinch salt

¾ tsp baking soda

2 apples, peeled and chopped

1-1/2 cup rolled oats

20 unwrapped caramel candies

2 tbsp water

Preheat oven to 325 degrees F.

In a large mixing bowl, use a mechanical mixer on medium speed to beat brown sugar and butter until creamy.

Add milk, egg, and vanilla, and beat for 2 minutes to fluff.

In a large, separate bowl, combine baking soda with flour and salt. Whisk to mix, then stir in oats.

Add dry mixture to wet mixture while beating on low speed.

When blended, stir in apples by hand.

Drop cookies onto baking sheets and bake for 14 minutes.

Let cool.

In a small saucepan, melt caramels and water together for 7 minutes over low heat or until smooth.

Remove caramel sauce from heat and drizzle evenly over cookies. Let stand 15 minutes.

Serve.

Onion Dip

1 tbsp olive oil

1 head of garlic

2 peeled and quartered sweet onions

1 tsp salt

¼ cup chopped parsley

1/3 cup nonfat sour cream

1 tbsp lemon juice

Preheat oven to 425 degrees F.

In a large bowl, place onion wedges and drizzle with olive oil. Add salt and toss to coat well.

Remove skin from garlic and wrap in a small square of tin foil.

Place garlic and onion onto a baking sheet, and bake in oven for 1 hour.

Cool for 10 minutes, then unwrap garlic and chop together with onion.

Combine in a large bowl with sour cream, lemon juice, and parsley.

Cover and chill in refrigerator for 1 hour.

Serve.

Orange Muffins

½ cup cake flour

6 tbsp hazelnut flour

Pinch salt

1 tsp baking powder

2 tbsp 2% milk

2 tbsp canola oil

1-1/2 tbsp grated orange rind

1-1/2 tbsp agave nectar or organic honey

1 tbsp orange juice

1 lightly beaten egg

Preheat oven to 350 degrees F.

In a large bowl, combine baking powder with both flours and salt.

In a separate large bowl, combine milk with oil, agave, orange juice, orange rind, and egg with a whisk.

Add dry mixture to wet, and stir until just moist.

Spoon into muffin cups and bake for 12 minutes or until done in the centers.

Let cool, then serve.

Juicing

Bring these delicious juices on board when you are looking for a great diet supplement.

Pear Salad

1 head endive

1 pear

1 inch of ginger root

1 cucumber

½ lemon

1 zucchini

Peel lemon and wash all other vegetables.

Process through a juicer and enjoy!

Sweet Pink

2 carrots

¼ watermelon

¼ pineapple

2 stalks celery

2 inch of ginger root

Peel pineapple and cut into chunks. Do not use rind.

Leave rind on watermelon and wash all produce well.

Process through a juicer and enjoy!

Spicy Warmth

6 romaine lettuce leaves

¼ head green cabbage

1 inch of ginger root

½ cucumber

1 pear

4 pieces of fresh mint

Slice cabbage into wedges and remove stems from pear and mint.

Wash all produce.

Process through a juicer and enjoy!

Red Red Juice

1 cup fresh spinach

4 chard sprigs, leaves and stems included

2 oranges

1 beet with leaves

1 lemon

1 inch piece turmeric root

Peel oranges, lemon, and beet before using.

Wash all produce.

Process through a juicer and enjoy!

Good Morning

1 orange

1 grapefruit

2 carrots

½ inch piece ginger root

Peel grapefruit and orange before using.

Wash all produce.

Process through a juicer and enjoy!

Warm Autumn

1 pear

1 beet

4 collar leaves

5 carrots

3 stalks of celery

1 inch piece ginger root

Peel beet and remove stems from collard leaves and pear

Wash all produce.

Process through a juicer and enjoy!

Florida Summer

2 lemons

2 oranges

1 grapefruit

½ inch of turmeric root

Peel lemon, orange, and grapefruit.

Wash all produce.

Process through a juicer and enjoy!

Sample One-Week Meal Plan

Try this meal plan in order to get your diet off on the right foot! Many of the meals included in this plan can be prepared ahead of time and either reheated or enjoyed cold when it comes time to eat. If you have a little bit of extra time on the weekend before you get started on your 41-day challenge, consider making some of your meals and putting them up in the refrigerator or freezer so that your week can be that much easier!

Remember to follow this meal plan along with the weekly workout plan listed in a previous chapter in order to start your diet off correctly. Keep following a similar meal plan throughout the rest of your 41 weeks and you will see the weight fall off fast!

Monday

Breakfast: Yogurt Parfait

Lunch: BLT

Dinner: Cumin Chicken

Snack: Orange Muffins

Juice: Good Morning

Tuesday

Breakfast: Scrambler

Lunch: Spelt Bean Salad

Dinner: Easy Chili

Snack: Homemade Hummus

Juice: Warm Autumn

Wednesday

Breakfast: Banana Bread

Lunch: Curry Chicken Salad

Dinner: Barbecue Chicken Potato

Snack: Orange Muffins

Juice: Spicy Warmth

Thursday

Breakfast: Yogurt Parfait

Lunch: Leftover Barbecue Chicken Potato

Dinner: Stuffed Chile Poblanos

Snack: Caramel Cookie Bites

Juice: Sweet Pink

Friday

Breakfast: Banana Bread

Lunch: Pasta Salad

Dinner: Tropical Ham Quesadillas

Snack: Quick Guacamole

Juice: Red Red Juice

Saturday

Breakfast: Avocado Muffin Sandwich

Lunch: Avocado Soup

Dinner: Grilled Chops

Snack: Caramel Cookie Bites

Juice: Florida Summer

Sunday

Breakfast: Poached Eggs

Lunch: Leftover Grilled Chops

Dinner: Wine Glazed Scallops

Snack: Onion Dip

Juice: Pear Salad

Conclusion

Are you ready to lose weight fast and stay in shape easily? Have you decided that it is finally time to make an important change in your life? By following my simple diet and exercise plan, you will be able to lose weight in 41 days and keep it off for as long as you like. You will be ready to show off your new, thinner body the next time you go to the beach, and you are sure to have a figure you are proud of, no matter what size you are to begin with!

By following my diet plan and preparing the many healthy recipes provided for you in the previous pages, you will have no trouble enjoying delicious, light foods that are easy to make in no time. You will even be able to serve these meals and delicious juices to your friends and family, all without ever mentioning that you are on a diet plan! When you incorporate the tasty juices and amazing meals into your daily routine and add in a few simple workouts throughout the week, you will find yourself losing weight faster than you ever could have imagined.

So, are you ready to feel amazing and discover how the diet and exercise plan that worked for me can make your life better as well? Join me in weight loss today, and see for yourself how this 41-day challenge can make you feel better and look great just in time for bikini season!

-- Lewis Green

www.ingramcontent.com/pod-product-compliance
Lightning Source LLC
Chambersburg PA
CBHW050758290526
45792CB00008B/2241